Your Fitness Training 2-in-1

Yoga Poses and Calisthenics for Beginners

Timothy Morrison

Table of Content

Your Fitness Training 2-in-1 1

Table of Content..2

Preface to the Second Edition...4

Calisthenics for Beginners: 5

Introduction 6

Step 1: Choose the Right Strength Training Exercises According to Your Fitness Level. 8

You Can't Do Pull-ups? Then This Chapter is for You! 12

Step 2: Apply Bodybuilding Training Principles to Your Workout. 14

Step 3: Learn About Full-body Workout and Split Training Routine. 16

Step 4: Improve Your Cardiovascular Fitness. 20

Step 5: Don't Forget About Recovery. 25

Step 6: Sleep Better, Rehab Faster. 26

Step 7: Stick to a Muscle-Building Diet.......................................28

Step 8: Use Periodized Training Plans for Better Results. 30

Step 9: Set SMART Fitness Goals...32

Step 10: Track Your Progress Using a Training Diary. 34

Conclusion...35

Yoga Poses Benefits of Yoga Practice According to Yoga Sutras of Patanjali 37

Introduction 38

Classical Yoga Centers around Patanjali's Yoga Sutras. 42

Benefits of Yoga Practice 43

General Guidelines 45

Asana 47

Corpse Pose (Savasana) 50

Seated Forward Bend (Paschimottanasana) 52

Cobra Pose (Bhujangasana) 54

Locust Pose (Salabhasana) 56

Shoulder stand (Sarvangasana) 58

Plow Pose (Halasana) 60

Bow Pose (Dhanurasana) 61

Hero Pose (Virasana) 62

Boat Pose (Navasana) 64

Downward-Facing Dog (Adho Mukha Svanasana) 66

Chair Pose (Utkatasana) 67

Eagle Pose (Garudasana) 68

Extended Side Angle (Utthi Parsvakonasana) 70

Tree Pose (Vrksasana) 72

Conclusion 73

Preface to the Second Edition

Hello! I'm Timothy Morrison and first of all I want to thank you for taking the time to purchase this book; I hope you'll enjoy reading it! This bundle consists of two manuscripts.

The first of them is "**Calisthenics for beginners: 10 steps to build your own bodyweight training program**"

And the second thing is "**Yoga poses: the benefits of yoga practice according sutras of Patanjali**"

These two books are completely different and at the same time they complement each other nicely. Both books provide you with knowledge about effective physical practice in order to disclose your potential.

Calisthenics provide effective workouts for your muscles. And yoga is more about relaxation and recovery for your mind and body.

Surely some styles of yoga like Ashtanga are physically demanding and look like good aerobic workout. Moreover, some yoga asana are very similar to gymnastic exercises. For instance, Wheel or Bridge exercise is known as Chakrasana in yoga.

However, I have a different vision for yoga. I like to think about yoga practice as meditative practice and a resource for fast recovery after hard workouts. As we know, we can't progress in our strength training without proper rehabilitation. That's why I consider yoga and calisthenics as two halves of the whole workout-recovery system; they just like Yin and Yang of our fitness training.

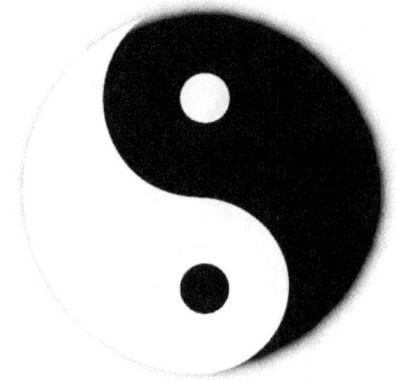

Calisthenics for Beginners:

10 Steps to Build Your Own Bodyweight Training Program

Combine the Best Bodyweight Exercises in Ways that Allow You to get an Incredibly Effective Street Workout

Introduction

The word calisthenics comes from the ancient Greek words kalos (κάλλος), which means "beauty", and sthenos (σθένος), meaning "strength". It is the art of using one's body weight and qualities of inertia as a means to develop one's physique.
Wikipedia

Calisthenics has its origin in ancient times. Obviously, it was a sufficient component of warrior's and athlete's training since those old times. All basic bodyweight exercises like push-ups, squats, and pull-ups are as aged as man's first try at becoming stronger by virtue of physical training.

And ironically, Calisthenics also is one of the **newest** trends in the fitness world. Term 'Calisthenics' is closely connected with 'street workout.' There are few worldwide sports organizations like the World Street Workout & Calisthenics Federation (WSWCF) and World Calisthenics Organization (WCO). Rules for competitions with judging criteria and weight categories are created too.

As we see generally, Calisthenics is associated with bodyweight strength training and gymnastic tricks on an overhand bar and parallel bars.

However, I believe that Calisthenics is something much wider than that. It is closer to the physical development term. Besides the strength, you should develop your endurance, your coordination, your dexterity, your balance.

Also, bodyweight exercise is an umbrella term for some disciplines that use gravity and inertia of body as a primary form of resistance. For instance, yoga and gymnastics are well known and very popular disciplines. Parkour is another example that has increased in popularity of late. Some experts consider cardiovascular exercise like running to be forms of bodyweight exercise too.

You are the person who defines the goals and builds your own system of training. Changing with time your aims and priorities is a quite natural way of your physical development. You also could choose a set of skills which is a key factor in your favorite sport and work on it.

Don't afraid to try something new and define what works for you. The dogmatic approach doesn't work well in long term perspective. The best training plan is the one you are going to follow up.

The more you train in new ways and angles, the easier it becomes to gain new skills. On the other hand, you need some time and efforts to progress in one particular direction. The balance between your goals and your time plus efforts is a key factor here. You should remember that.

Step 1: Choose the Right Strength Training Exercises According to Your Fitness Level.

As we admitted previously, bodyweight exercises are known for centuries if not longer. However, the ways these exercises are performed are also developing rapidly. Training schemes, principles, and programs now draw heavily from weightlifting bodybuilding which is a mainstream way to add strength and gain muscle. The great thing about weight lifting and bodyweight training is that you don't have to pick one or the other. Mix up the type of stimulation. It's a good way to shock your muscles into new growth incessantly.

Bodyweight exercises imitate real life moves. You probably have heard a "functional training" term. So you learn to be strong and to perform in ways you will need to in real life. That's why Calisthenics is good for conditioning for sports such as boxing or martial arts.

Basic exercises in Calisthenics are compound movements. It is convenient to divide all muscle groups to upper body muscles and lower body muscles. Upper body muscles in their turn could be split into two another groups: push and pull.

Push muscles primarily include chest, shoulders, and triceps. It is logical that main movements here are push-ups and dips. Actually, they are two variants of one movement.

Regular **push-ups** are simple and handy exercises, require nothing more than the floor beneath your feet. If you don't have access to weight-training equipment, you still can perform push-ups. The proper form of push-ups provides the load for your entire core, not just your upper body.

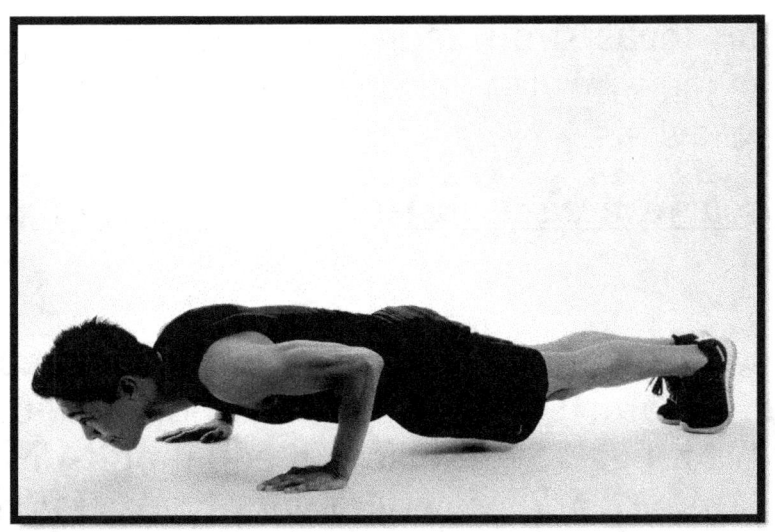

There is a huge number of push-ups variants with different levels of difficulty. Most challenging are one hand push-ups and headstand push-ups. You'll need not only a sufficient level of strength but also a significant amount of stability for performing headstand push-ups. One hand push-ups force you to engage your lats, opposite-side leg, lower back, and glutes.

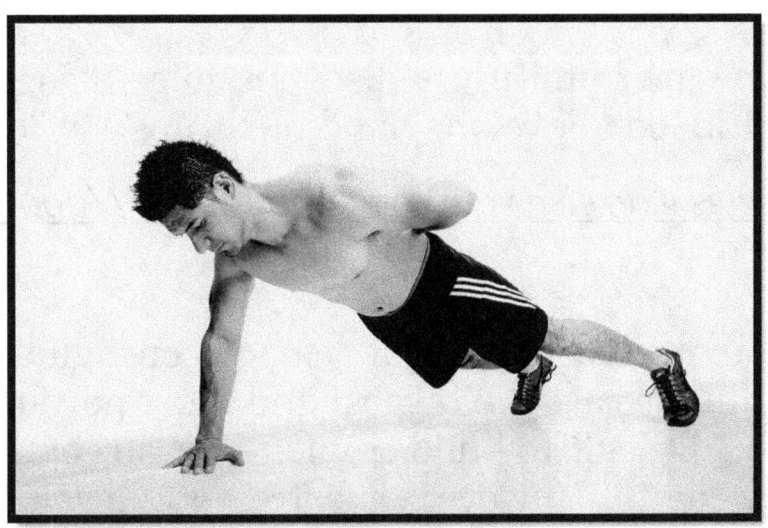

The **dip** is another old-school, simple-yet-brutally-effective exercise. It is just one of the best exercises you can perform to explode your chest, shoulders, and triceps. Parallel bar dips train your push muscles in an entirely different angle than push-ups and bench pressing.

You also could try ring dips. Such form requires much more stability to perform. It's one of the harder variations you can do.

We are not focused on details of exercise's technique in this book. Training videos work perfectly, so I have added some links to YouTube playlists.

Push muscles exercises on YouTube: https://goo.gl/TRisUP

Pull muscles primarily include back and biceps. Apparently, this body part is trained by **pull-ups**. Pull-up is a gold standard exercise for back training. No exercise can equal pull-ups for effectiveness in building strength and growth of your back. It is the fact that in gyms many people prefer to use pull-down machines than pull-ups. Not surprisingly, many gym-goers are unable of doing even one clean pull-up. Invest your time and efforts to be strong at pull-ups. It will develop real strength, muscle mass, and explosiveness.

There is also a wide variety of different ways to execute pull-ups. For example, you can use wide or close grip. Underhand grip is another option here.

A true one-arm pull-up is also possible. It is tough, much harder than mentioned above one hand push-ups.

Pull muscles exercises on YouTube: https://goo.gl/XMMEEY

Lower body primarily includes quadriceps, glutes, and calves. Some of these muscles are the biggest and most powerful in your body. So, it could be difficult to build tremendous strength in your lower body without weights. However, if extremely developed leg muscles are not paramount to you, then do not worry about it. Bodyweight squats, lunges and different kinds of jumps work well here.

And, of course, one leg **pistol squats** come to mind as a most challenging variant. As some others Calisthenics exercise pistol develops the perfect combination of power, balance, coordination, and flexibility.

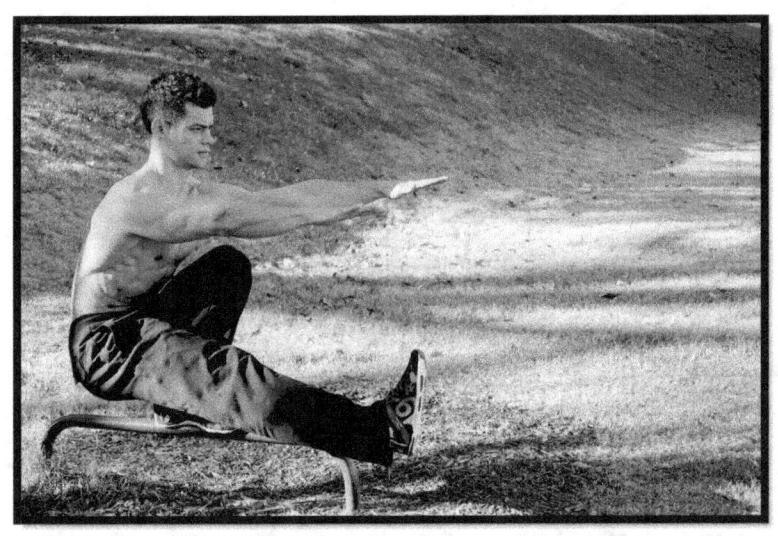

Leg exercises on YouTube: https://goo.gl/R2Tnu0

Beyond that, abs are trained by leg raising, sit-ups, crunches.

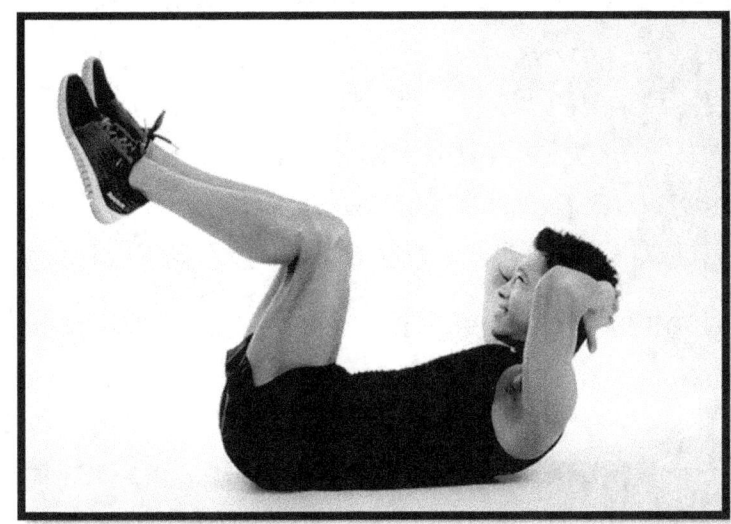

Plank works excellent for the whole core. A well-developed core shows both power and health. The hyperextension on the ground keeps in tone your low back.

Core exercises on YouTube: https://goo.gl/k5dba2

So, pull-ups are hard. Surely, you might be not very good at them, especially, if you're just started. Then it is reasonable to consider making your back exercises a priority number 1 in your training plan. There are few exercises which are perfect precursors to regular pull ups. It's also a good cause to learn some of the hypertrophy training principles.

1.   Horizontal pull-ups are also known under name 'reverse push-ups.' This variation is a lot easier since your weight is on the floor mostly. Still, it's a good first step to the vertical, usual pull-up.

An isometric exercise is a form of exercise involving the static contraction of a muscle without any visible movement in the angle of the joint. The term "isometric" combines the Greek words "Isos" (equal) and "metria" (measuring), meaning that in these exercises the length of the muscle and the angle of the joint do not change, though contraction strength may be varied.

2.   Timed hang or 'dead hang' is an isometric exercise. Hang with straight arms and feet of the ground for 10-30 seconds or as long as you can. Focus on keeping your shoulders in the packed position. Don't let them up around your neck. You can use different grip variations in following sets.

3.   The static hold is also hanging on the bar but this time on the top movement of the pull-up. You hold that flexed position for 10-30 seconds or as long as you can.

A negative repetition (negative rep) is the repetition of a technique in weightlifting in which the lifter performs the eccentric phase of a lift. Instead of pressing the weight up slowly, in proper form, a spotter generally aids in the concentric, or lifting, portion of the repetition while the lifter slowly performs the eccentric phase for 3–6 seconds. Negative reps are used to improve both muscular strength and power.

4.   Negative pull-ups are half pull-ups. From the top position, you lower yourself down slowly, in-control. How to set up that top position? There are a set of options. You can use a bench, or a box, or a chair. You can jump above the pull bar or use a help of your training partner.

Partial reps, as the name implies, involves movement through only part of the normal path of an exercise. Partial reps can be performed with heavier weights. Usually, only the easiest part of the repetition is attempted.

5.   Partial pull-ups involve only partial amplitude – at the top or the bottom of a movement. Top-partial pull-ups are my favorite, but you should try both variants. You also can do partial reps after complete pull-ups, when you can't do any more full reps.

As you can see, pull-ups mastering is all about progressions. I mean a chain of exercises that get progressively more difficult until you rich your goal. And off cause you can't do pull-ups if you don't practice pull-ups. So, it's up to you.

Pull-up tips for beginners on YouTube: https://goo.gl/VpXGlp

Step 2: Apply Bodybuilding Training Principles to Your Workout.

In the previous chapter we have considered such training principles as negatives, partial reps, and isometric tension. There are many other advanced techniques. Most of them were gathered and honed by Joe Weider, the father of modern bodybuilding.

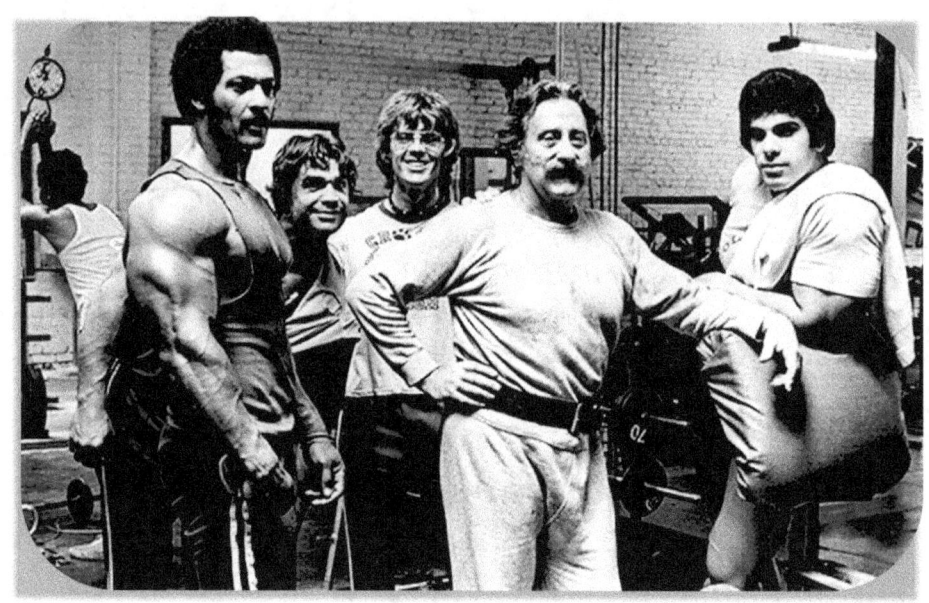

Some of that principles work to bodyweight training perfectly.

Push-pull supersets pair exercises for opposing body parts in sequence without rest. In bodybuilding gyms, this method is especially popular when applied to arm training. Arnold used supersets to his chest-back workout mostly. You can do both by combination pull-ups and dips. You allow your chest and triceps to rehab while your back and biceps are working, and vice versa. So, you can do more repetition in each set. As a result, you'll get a sizable pumping, and that visual benefit is superb motivation. You also can do a lot of work in short time. On the hormonal level, push-pull superset leads to a spike of HGH, which is responsible for muscle growth and fat loss.

Supersets of exercises for the same body part are much more exhausting. For example, you can combine dips with push-ups. Another variant is pull-ups with 'reverse push-ups.' Regular squats after pistol squats are also good for your legs.

Forced reps are repetition after your muscular failure. You will need a training partner who provides enough help to complete the set. It's a classic thing with pull-ups. It is also applicable with dips.

The **rest-pause** method could be implemented in two options.

1.   You take your set to failure, then rest for 10-20 seconds, and continue to do reps till you reach failure once more. Repeat this trick 2-3 times per set and you will get more reps in a given exercise.

2.   You choose an exercise that only allows you to get 3-5 repetitions. You do one rep, rest 15 seconds, and perform another rep. Your goal is 4-6 repetitions, which form one rest-pause set. This variant is effective at increasing muscle strength.

Step 3: Learn About Full-body Workout and Split Training Routine.

How often should you do your strength training? Well, the answer depends on too many factors. I like to train each muscle group twice a week. One of the workouts is hard, and another is light.

On the hard training, I try to push my limits by increasing number of reps or/and sets. Using some of the principles described in the previous chapter is possible too.

The light training is just refreshing for muscles, and you don't need many sets and reps. You should focus on proper technique instead. You can also try some new exercise or method during your light training.

For example, my previous hard and light training plans for pull muscles look like:

Monday, hard training.

1. Wide-grip pull-ups, 5 sets of 10 reps.

Usually, the last set is challenging one. I can do 7 to 8 repetitions before reaching failure. Then I do from 1 to 3 forced reps. Use the box to help yourself to bring your chin over the bar.

2. Wide-grip reverse push-ups on the low horizontal bar, 2 sets of 20 reps.

Keep the negative phase of movement lasted twice as the positive one.

3. Dead hang, one set for as long as possible.

I've found that my grip is the weak link in the chain of pull muscles. Train your forearms to progress faster in pull-ups.

Thursday, light training.

1. Middle-grip pull-ups, 3 sets of 5 reps.

Focus on the strict technique of your movements. Besides, my back and biceps are still in pain after the hard training on Monday.

2. Close-grip chin-ups, 3 sets of 5 reps.

I like this form with the accent on my biceps. Probably, I'll include chin-ups in my hard training later.

Full body workout combines exercises like push-ups, pull-ups, basic core work, and squats. This style of training twice per week can build strength without sacrificing hours to the gym. Full body is one of the oldest and well-known training plans.

	Monday (Tuesday)	Thursday (Friday)
Push muscles	HARD	LIGHT
Pull muscles	LIGHT	HARD
Legs	HARD	LIGHT
Core	LIGHT	HARD

You train all your muscles per workout; you have enough time for recovery. Full body scheme works quite well any goal like increasing strength, building muscle, losing fat.

Upper-lower body training split is the next level. You are training four times per week now: two upper body workouts and two lower body workouts. You do all chosen kinds of pull-ups, dips, and push-ups on your upper body workout. Lower body workout includes squats, jumps, exercises for your core and lower back. Upper-lower body split allows you to spend more time and efforts on every muscle group. Mentioned above push-pull supersets fit perfectly. You still train each muscle group twice a week. And you still mix hard and light training days.

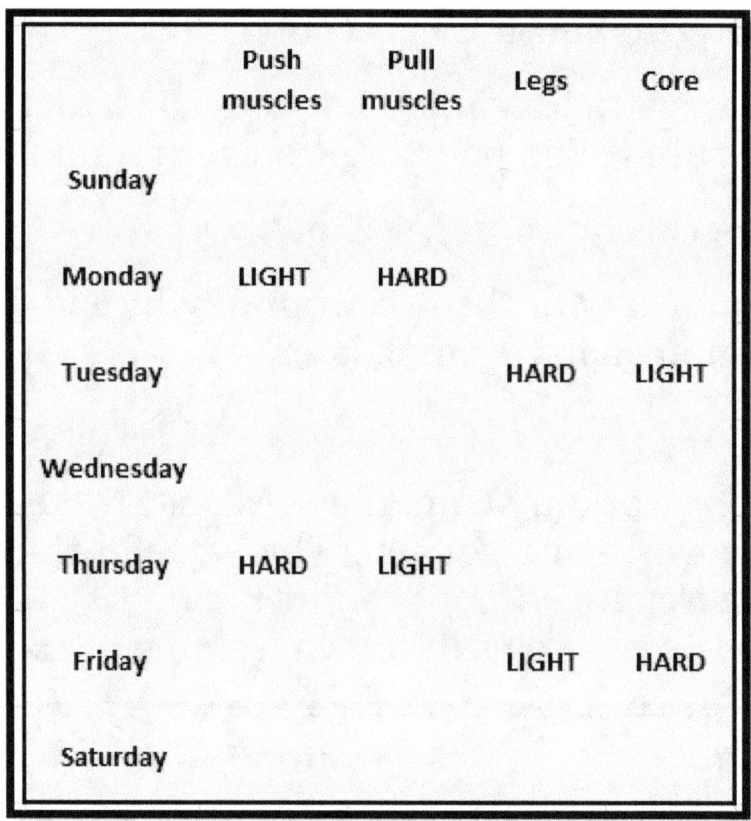

	Push muscles	Pull muscles	Legs	Core
Sunday				
Monday	LIGHT	HARD		
Tuesday			HARD	LIGHT
Wednesday				
Thursday	HARD	LIGHT		
Friday			LIGHT	HARD
Saturday				

Here is an example of an upper-lower body split training plan. To perform a superset, execute exercises with the same digit but different letter designation back to back, without rest between them. Rest interval between supersets is 60 seconds.

Monday: pull hard, push light.

1A. Wide-grip pull-ups, 5 sets of 12 reps.

1B. Pike push-ups, 5 sets of 10 reps.

2A. Close-grip, chin-ups, 3 sets of 8 reps.

2B. Dips on bench, 3 sets of 8 reps.

Tuesday: legs hard, core light.

1.   Pistol squats, 5 sets of 12 reps.

2.   Jump squats, 4 sets of 20 reps

3A. Crunches, 3 sets of 25 reps

3B. Reverse crunches, 3 sets of 25 reps.

Thursday: push hard, pull light

1A. Dips on parallel bars, 5 sets of 15 reps

1B. Horizontal pull-ups, 5 sets of 15 reps.

2A. Knuckle push-ups, 3 sets of 20 reps.

2B. Dead hang, 3 sets. Try last for 60 seconds each set.

Friday: core hard, legs light.

1.   Legs raises on pull-up bar, 5sets of 15 reps.

2A. High crunches, 3 sets of 20 reps.

2B. Floor hyperextensions, 3 sets of 20 reps.

3.   Plank, for 60 seconds.

4A. Lunges, 5 sets of 15 reps.

4B. Squats, 5 sets of 20 reps.

Don't forget to change exercise with time. Try new variants on your light days. Then implement them in your hard training.

Pull-push-legs split provides even more focus for every muscle group of yours. Pulling muscles, pushing muscles, and legs are trained separately on their own workout day. There are six workouts in a week. And still, every muscle group is worked roughly twice per week and allowed roughly 72 hours to rehab.

Step 4: Improve Your Cardiovascular Fitness.

Cardio also is known as aerobic exercise is a physical activity that is long, repetitive, and depends mostly on the aerobic metabolism. Cardio in some way is opposite to anaerobic (strength) training. The difference is in duration and intensity of work. For instance, jogging is a cardio drill, though sprinting is an anaerobic exercise.

Several studies show us that cardio training can elevate results of strength training. With cardiovascular exercises, you will get greater gains! For instance, cardio can boost your work capacity during bodyweight strength workout; enhance your recovery between sessions, and improve your muscular physique. As we know, in order to burn fat and slim down, some amount of cardio training will need to be done.

Systematic prolonged training stimulates the growth of new blood vessels in your muscles. As a result, your muscle tissue gets more oxygen, macro- and micronutrients, vitamins, and therefore repairs faster.

It is also possible to strengthen your heart with regular cardio exercise. Indeed, doing aerobic exercises over the years, you can develop your heart in volume. And heart's work becomes more efficient in this case.

Good aerobic workout makes you feel like a totally new person. You know that feeling of lightness and freedom, and your mind becomes clear. After forty minutes of intense cardio training, your body starts to regenerate your nerve cells. New neurons begin to appear too. Surprisingly, the old and well-known expression 'nerve cells do not regenerate' doesn't work for you anymore.

In order to achieve the best possible result of training, you need to pick an exercise that fit your purpose. And again the best choice is the one you are going to stick with. Surely, you can change your exercises depending on the target and mood. The basic rule here is 'don't give up training.' If you want to have a stable and long-term effect, you must regularly train throughout the life. Without training sessions, all health benefits will disappear in a few weeks.

Cardio training is not just about running and rope skipping; the same old cardio gets boring very quickly. Cardio training includes numerous different exercises. The biggest part of them is performed chiefly by the leg muscles. However, there are some exceptions. What is your favorite sport to watch? Which is your favorite sport to play? The more you train your muscles and brain in new and foreign ways, the easier it becomes to master new skills. Basketball, tennis, baseball, and football places far greater demands on coordination, balance, and flexibility than strength training alone does.

If you like boxing and other martial arts you should take a look at Tae Bo. This fitness system was invented and developed by Billy Blanks. Tae Bo combines aerobic exercises, kicks, and punches. Actually, the name 'Tae Bo' goes from taekwondo and boxing.

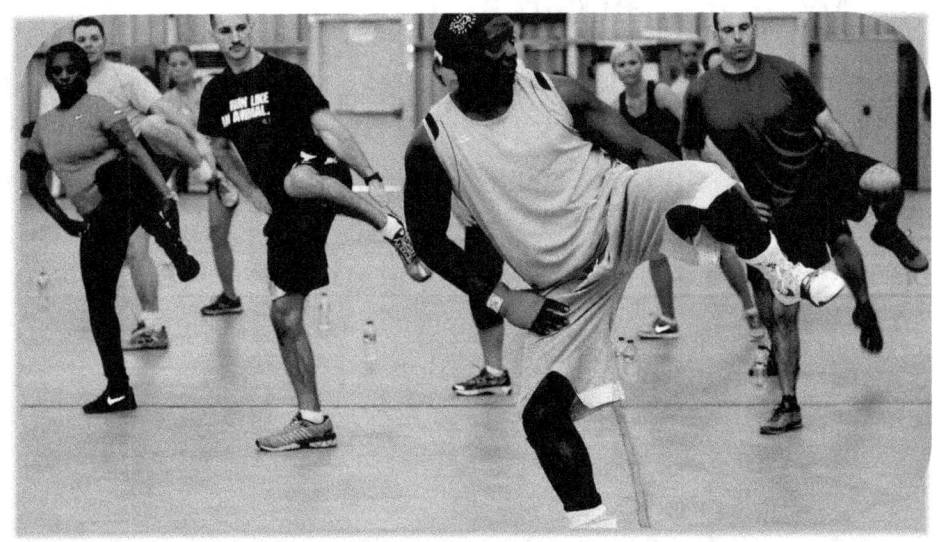

Though Tae Bo is not intended for combat or self-defense, your fight part of 'fight-or-flight' instinct could be encouraged sufficiently. Finding such a 'deep reason' creates a strong motivation for your training. The best training plan is the one you are going stick to, remember? If you enjoy what you are doing, you will progress very fast.

Personally, I've found that shadowboxing fits me just perfectly. Shadow-boxing is the practice of performing repetitive fighting movements to muscle memory. Clearly, it works well for striking techniques, not for grappling. Shadowboxing is one of the most important drills to improve technique, speed, endurance, rhythm, footwork, defense and offense, and overall fighting abilities. The primary goal here is to get used to fighting movements. This exercise is pure calisthenics as soon as you don't need any equipment. Shadowboxing is also completely harmless as there is no opponent trying to hit you.

Shadowbox according to rounds. You should plan each round before you start shadowbox. Trying to work on every aspect at once is the worst thing you can do for your progress. So, you need a goal.

If your goal is **warming-up** use shadowboxing to get warm and break a sweat. Use footwork actively, don't forget about head-movement, and throw punches. Keep your body in motion. Move designedly in, out, and around.

Shadowboxing is the best of acquiring proper **technique**. This exercise should be used to habituate each new move like a punch, defensive tech, or footwork. Repetitions are necessary but only after you know that you are doing right. I mean, you need feedback. This is where having someone more experienced in boxing helps. Also, it is a good idea to practice in front of a full-length mirror so that the movements can be watched for correct form.

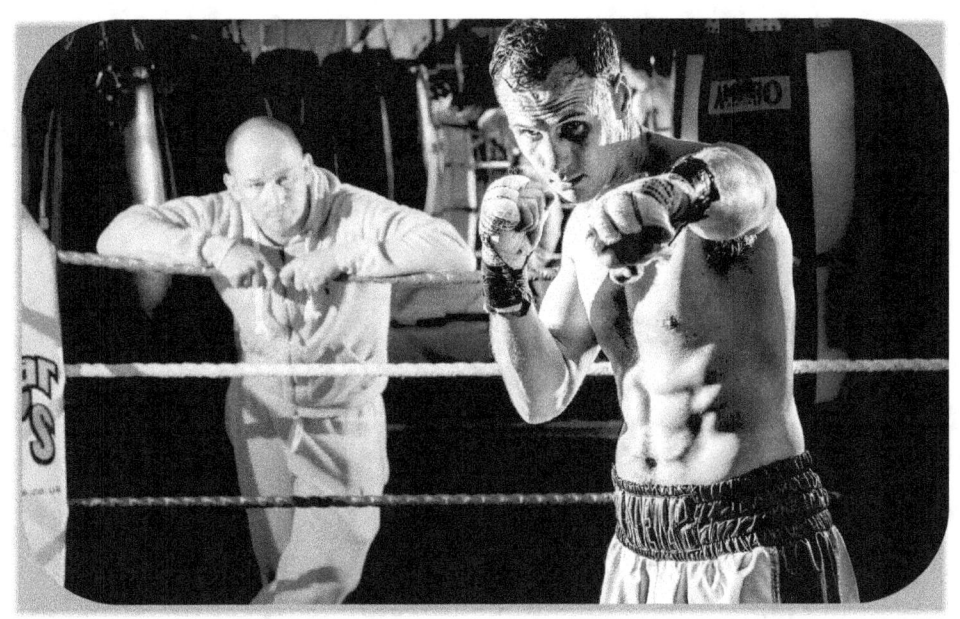

One more reason to shadowbox is developing your **coordination** and **balance**. Every time you are training you work on developing new mind-muscle connections. Eventually, during a real fight or intense sparring, this is what you will rely on. Your rival always tries to make you miss, and in every miss you get off-balanced. Shadowboxing is the perfect method to train the supporting muscles to counteract the momentum generated in every your attack. After all, with well developed stabilizing muscles and coordination, you can throw nice combos of powerful shots while maintaining balanced.

Simulating actual actions used in a fight will **condition** your hand and leg endurance. You also can work on your **rhythm** while shadowboxing by making many punches, defenses, and footwork. Throwing punches with full extension and power all the time is not a very good idea for your joint health. So sometimes it is ok to minimize your hand movements. Let's focus on torso rotation over arm extension, and your joints will thank you for it. Explosive footwork and head movement will provide sufficient level of intensity.

Shadowboxing is a mental exercise also. You could go into every round with focus on implementing specific **strategies**. And yes, strategies are needed even for something as primary as fighting. Shadowboxing is an excellent opportunity to work out a strategy to beat your opponent. Then you master new technical things like punch combinations to fulfill this plan. Punches are often labeled with digits to simplify training process. There are typical numbers associated with every punch in boxing:

1 – jab

2 – right straight (cross)

3 – left hook

4 – right hook (overhand)

5 – left uppercut

6 – right uppercut

Body shots are just called as 'body'. Basic punching combinations are:

1-2   with variations (1 – 2body,   1body – 2)

1 – 2 – 3   (1 – 2body – 3,   1 – 2 – 3body,   1body – 2 – 3)

1 – 1 – 2   (1 – 1 – 2body,   1 – 1body – 2,   1body – 1 – 2)

1 – 2 – 1   (1body – 2 – 1,   1 – 2body – 1)

1 – 2 – 3 – 2   (1 – 2body – 3 – 2, 1body – 2 – 3 – 2)

Master the standard punch combo. Then try advanced or/and start creating your own. Surely, with the kicks, elbows, and knees in your arsenal, you will have an even much wider diversity of your training routine. *Examples of shadowboxing routines on YouTube: https://goo.gl/TYDo8q*

Shadowboxing also could be substituted in place of an aerobic or anaerobic conditioning session, with the duration and intensity reflecting a jogging for long distance or set of sprints.

Step 5: Don't Forget About Recovery.

The whole training process and its benefits are all about keeping the balance between stress and recovery. Due to strength exercise execution, you break some part of your muscle tissue down. After a workout, your muscle fibers repair themselves and come back bigger and stronger than they were before. As you can see, the scheme of the whole process is pretty simple. The tricky part is to define how much time you need to recover efficiently. Because, if you tax the same muscles every day heavily, you aren't them the time they need to rehab. As a result, you'll get overtraining. Usual signals of overtraining are decreased performance, elevated blood pressure, decreased immunity, disturbed sleep.

By performing hard-light workout scheme and training splits, you train each muscle group enough to add strength, but not so much that you need to rest for too many days between each strength workout. Plus, you have time to enjoy your cardio training on a more recreational basis. Such an active recovery will provide the blood flowing, more nutrients, and oxygen to those sore, torn muscles. Naturally, this will accelerate the process of recovery.

To determine adequate rest between workouts you should consider many different factors. Your age could be a factor and how intensely you train, how often you work out, and the duration of exercise.

So, you will listen to your body and change your schedule when you need. For example, if you feel sore for hard-day strengthen workout, perform cardio or light-day session. Yes, light training is one of the best ways to resolve muscle soreness. This phenomenon is well known as 'repeated-bout effect.'

Or, if you feel exhausted all of the time, you may need to take one more day off. Probably, you like many people tend to over-train, which can delay your progress. You should keep symptoms of overtraining at bay. It's all about maintaining balance, remember?

The best training routine, diet and supplement plan will not compensate for poor quality sleep. Sleep just might be the most important element of your training schedule. Often the key to winning is the quality and amount of sleep you get. You need at least eight hours of quality sleep per night. Elite athletes are known to sleep ten hours a night and nap throughout the day between workouts to maintain their endurance. 'Get enough for you' is the best practical recommendation here.

Little sleep means little results because without adequate rest your body will fail to adapt. Of course, you can be sleep deprived from time to time. However, if it is a permanent situation, it will have an enormous impact on your training results. Also, getting too little sleep accumulates a so-called 'sleep debt.' We couldn't adapt to getting less sleep than we need, so your body will 'pay back,' eventually.

Sleep has a profound effect on physical well-being and every part of our life. Up to 70% of daily human growth hormone secretion is naturally released under conditions of sleep. This hormone stimulates fat burning, muscle growth, and repair. Thus the more sleep you get, the faster your body will heal and recover from exercise.

Your exercise can help your sleep; it is kind of synergy effect. However, sometimes it is hard to get a good night of sleep. The following simple rules can assist in getting that proper night rest.

Complete your training at least four hours before going to bed. Avoid caffeine and other stimulants within those four hours too. Don't eat large meals just before bedtime, small snacks are allowed.

Go to bed and wake up at the consistent times every day.

Do not watch TV in bed, instead make some sleep routine. Shut off electronics and write in a diary. Take a warm bath. Minimize light and noise, meditate. Any other things that relax and bring down the body are acceptable.

Step 7: Stick to a Muscle-Building Diet.

Second, the most important recovery factor is food. You should focus on proper nutrition when it comes to getting the results you want. Intensive training is an incredibly demanding job. That's why what you ingest in the minutes and hours after your workout is so critical to recovery. One of the most beneficial things you can do for your calisthenics program is a post-workout nutrition strategy.

Ingesting carbohydrates within thirty minutes of the workout is crucial to initiating muscle glycogen synthesis. Experts recommend post-workout consuming 0.5g of carbs per pound of bodyweight.

Also, most experts agree that athletes will get hoped-for benefit by consuming right dose (30g) of protein within the first-hour post-workout.

Usually, we finish a training session in some fluid deficit. Drinking 150% of the estimated fluid loss will enhance rapid and complete recovery from dehydration. Sipping fluids is preferable to drinking large amounts at one time.

If you want to gain some muscle mass, you will need an excess of calories. If you are a teenage hard-gainer, you will need to consume even more calories because your metabolism is very high. When you take in more than expanded calories, and weight is being gained, fatigue reducing becomes much more efficient. You also eat much more carbs, up to 3g per pound per day for hard-training days.

During fat loss dieting you reduce consumption of carbohydrates, as well as calories intake. Keep in mind, that cutting carbs will have an adverse impact on fatigue. So, cut the minimum you can to get still the result you need. And make sure the other recovery factors like proper training management and quality sleep are in order.

As much as possible avoid junk food in favor of eating muscle building foods like white and red meat, whole eggs, and fish.

Vegetables and fruits contain not only carbohydrates but water, vitamins, minerals, antioxidants, and fiber. Some of these nutrients affect the speed at which glucose releases into the bloodstream. That's why these products are recommended for sustained energy during the day.

As we said previously, it is important to focus on one particular goal for a period of time. It is also a good intention to switch it up to a different goal at the next period. You don't want always be working towards the same goal. It's too boring, and your mind needs a change of pace in order to keep you motivated enough. At the same time, your body needs time to recover from training in a given mode.

Yes, the 'goal' is a key word here. The two most common fitness goals are building muscle and fat loss. And of course, I want to get both at once. However, you will achieve better results if you include two different periods in your training plan.

In order to perform your 'leaning out' phase, you are going to add more cardio in your program. You can start with two full-body strength workouts and four half-hour cardio sessions every week. You may also wish to make some changes in your diet. Moderation your calories and especially carbohydrates intake is a good move. You need clean sources of complex carbohydrates only, so avoid simple carbs. Timing is an important thing too. Cut down on your intake later on in the evening when your body needs less energy. Focus more on eating carbs in your breakfast and around your workout as this when you need fuel most. Be sure you are having lots of water.

In order to execute your 'gaining muscle' phase, you are going to focus on your strength workouts. I suppose four upper-lower-body split workouts and two cardio sessions a week is a good plan. You need many calories, and you should focus on clean sources of protein, carbs, and healthy fats at each meal.

How long should you stick to a particular phase? Well, I would say two to three months is an optimal duration. One excellent way to set up a training program is with seasons. Do you always try to lose fat come summer, like most people do? Then you can take this concept and build your program around it.

You are right; whole this periodization-thing looks like bodybuilders program, where they cycle periods of bulking with fat loss. Well, systematic planning of training applies in nearly all sports. Martial arts, wrestling, football, basketball, baseball, and swimming are a few that fall into this category. Actually, anyone interested in a general base of fitness, skills, and strength would, as well. These athletes would also require speed, strength endurance, hypertrophy, and aerobic endurance, to varying proportions. Each of these requires a special form of training and some conflict to the others. The common goal is preparation for the most important competition of the year. There are longer cycles for the Olympian, being four and eight years. Another example is the career plan which is usually only considered for professional athletes.

I couldn't stress enough the importance of having goals. Next crucial point in creating your bodyweight training program that will work best for you is figuring out what your fitness goal is. Whether you want to burn fat, increase strength or just look great naked adopting your training regimen plays a significant role.

Set goals for your nearest training cycle and apply the SMART criteria to each of your goals.

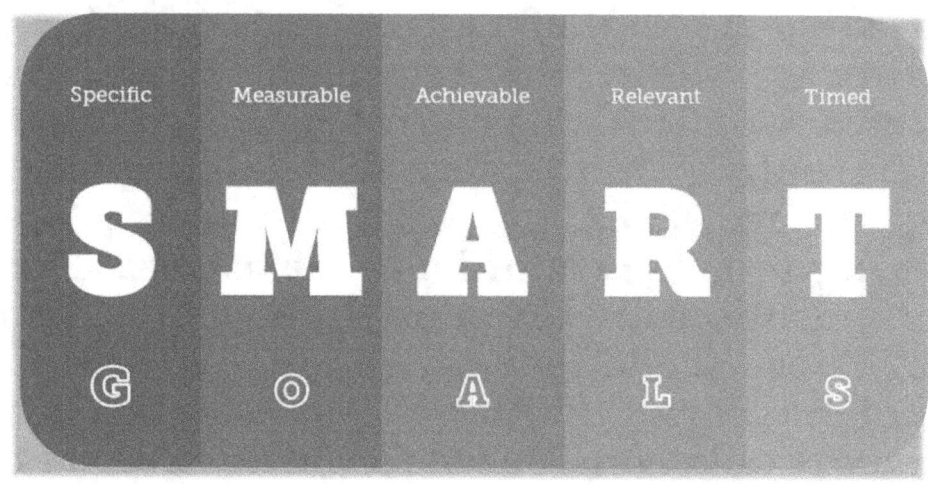

Specific aim declares exactly what you want to accomplish. For example, make a goal of 'performing ten reps of pistol squats' rather than 'increasing leg strength.'

Measurability allows you to track the progress and measure the outcome. How much muscle are you planning to gain? Put some numbers in your goal. These numbers could define exercise repetitions, fat percentage, waist to chest ratio, weight to gain, and so on.

Attainable goal is reasonable enough to be accomplished. If you have never done a single pull-up before, wanting to perform fifteen reps of regular pull-ups within a month is not an attainable goal. Obviously, you should always take into account your experience with certain exercise. Furthermore, after success with easier goals at the start, you will find yourself more motivated.

Relevant goal meets your need. If you want big arms, focus on exercises like chin-ups and bench dips. However, it is about your whole lifestyle, not only workouts. For instance, if you are unwilling to change your diet, then you can't expect to lose weight significantly in a couple of months.

Timed goal provides a time limit. It will establish a sense of urgency. Also, having a deadline will motivate you to stick to your program when you feel like slacking off. Eventually, setting a time limit will let you know whether or not you workout routine is effective as your progress.

Setting SMART goals do not have to be difficult, so let's give it a try. The summer is coming, and off course, I want six packs. I will know that I've achieved my purpose when I see a six-pack in the mirror. In order to realize my goal, I need to reduce body fat by five percent. I will do two strengthen workouts and four cardio sessions a week for the next two months. And I will increase my result in 'leg raises on bar' exercise by ten repetitions at the end of this cycle. I will cut my daily intake by 500 calories. I will avoid all kinds of sweetness and processed food. I will eat complex carbohydrates before and after my workouts. I won't drink a beer and sweet beverages, only plain water. I will stick to this regimen for the next two months.

It looks like I get a kit of goals, isn't it? Well, it happens when you want just to get six packs.

Step 10: Track Your Progress Using a Training Diary.

A training diary is one of the best tools you can use for achieving your goals; it's an important key to success. At its most basic minimum, this is a written record of exercises and repetitions for every set you do. Also, record the quality of your repetitions. I mean, if you did nine clean pull-ups and the tenth needed a tad of help, don't record all ten as if they all were done well. You should note the assisted repetition as only a half rep. If at one training session you rush between sets and then at the next session you take your time, you can't compare those two workouts evenly. You must be honest about details when entering data.

Indeed, your training diary should be more than just a list of exercises, sets, and reps. Many factors can be included in the journal. For instance, whether you intend to lose weight or not, monitoring your nutritional intake throughout the day is a reasonable move. In a few months, you will figure out the best foods to give you the best results.

If you are attempting to lose weight, it may be a good idea to monitor your body mass on a weekly basis. But please don't get into the useless habit of weighing yourself every day.

Also, record how many hours of sleep per night you are getting and how many times you wake in the night. Alternations in your sleep patterns may be a sign that your training load is too high.

Resting heart rate is a simple and workable indicator of your general physical wellbeing. A heart rate that's more than ten beats over your typical resting value is a sign of overtraining. But again, you need some stats.

Think of your training diary as a road map which is irreplaceable for keeping you on track for fitness success. With a detailed data, you will know what is working well for you and what doesn't. So, you can draw on when designing your future training programs.

Conclusion.

Fitness and general health are important parts of life. Good health is a result of a balanced lifestyle. Fitness should be a pleasant side of your life. There is nothing wrong with lifting weights. Actually, weights can be used for a variety of useful tricks. For example, you can pre-exhaust a particular muscle group before training a compound movement. I suppose it comes down to enjoying something and asking what you want from your workout. People who take up weight training usually more focused on building muscle mass and adding strength in certain movements. Calisthenics people are typically interested more in overall full-body strength than they are in increasing the size of isolated muscles. Both calisthenics and weight training contribute to general health and well-being. The best workout is the one that you actually will perform, remember?

Your real 'enemy at the gates' is a sedentary lifestyle. A sedentary lifestyle is a medical term used to describe a way of life with an excessive amount of daily sitting. Also, sedentary activities include lying, working the computer, watching TV, playing video games, and reading. Being inactive increases the risk of developing obesity, hypertension, cardiovascular disease, depression, anxiety, and premature aging.

Your genes, combined with your lifestyle choices, determine your health status. Our genes are virtually identical to those of our ancestors who lived here long ages ago. For them, daily physical activity was a necessary part of survival; it was not a lifestyle choice. In fact, today exercise is still essential for our general health and well-being. According to the Department of Health and Human Services, you need to be physically active for at least 150 minutes per week. Also, you should execute muscle-strengthening activities at least two days every week.

If you are sedentary, consult your physician before beginning any exercise regimen. It is never too late to make a change. Start with a light intensity aerobic activity that you enjoy. Gradually increase your level of activity each week until you reach optimal volume. Additionally to your aerobic exercise, start your muscle-strengthening program one day weekly, and gradually increase to more days.

So, calisthenics is about natural looking bodies, functional strength, building strong neurological connections to body, and creativity. Also, this is probably the most versatile of all workout styles. It seems that calisthenics is the future of fitness. By now it is evident there is a growing community of people who are committed to exercising with only the weight of their bodies and minimal equipment. You may join this community too!

Yoga Poses

Benefits of Yoga Practice According to Yoga Sutras of Patanjali

Introduction

"36.7 million Americans or 15% of US adults practice yoga in the US"

- From the report by Yoga Alliance about yoga in the US 2016.

The United States medical practitioners, as well as chiropractors, are concerned about the increasing amount of traumas which individuals end up getting at yoga training, particularly by the "high-speed" type also known as "power yoga" which comes into play increasingly more into fashion in the last years. Just as professionals remember, right now there had not recently been a growth very similar to that ever since the Eighties while Jane Fonda started off to promote aerobic exercise.

A couple of years ago, «Boston Globe» correspondents presented instances of "victims" eagerness for yoga training. As a result, a thirty-year individual was looking for operation after he got his knee joint damaged. A lady with broad knowledge of yoga exercise injured the neck after practice with a whole new "guru." One other guy destroyed a nerve and as a consequence lost responsiveness of his thigh.

Given that professionals recognize, in many instances, yoga exercise is less dangerous compared to several other techniques. Nevertheless, lots of people misunderstand it, switching it into contests, and even without preparatory coaching as well as necessary information results into accidental injuries.

To have an understanding of the advantages of yoga exercise, it's vital that you realize that it's not only stretching out. Yoga is larger, even if you don't include any particular spiritual or religious part into your practice.

Stress reducing is the benefit with a good number of testimonies. However, given that stress is a huge element in just about all facets of your overall health. Stress elimination is a worthy reward.

Nature is organized in such a way that time always operates against the life. Certainly one of the situations associated with the local order is a simple fact, which ultimately this order is depleted. The instant an individual is born, the deflection of life-support processes is continually accumulating. Doing yoga exercise can a lot slow down the standard rate of the entropy process. Yoga certainly influences the activity of immune system. It's not just invigorating, but setting immunity work gently. It permits yoga practice to be evenly useful both at immunodeficiency and also at autoimmune disease problems.

Yoga exercise is a step-by-step activity revitalizing the motion of the system to the order of a greater level. At the particular phase of this scheme, the relationship between the individual and his systemic mind happens to be optimized.

F. Capra («Tao of physics», 1975) previously had looked into many cultures as well as customs attempting to explain basic rules of well-being and longevity. He came to the conclusion that you have just 2 of them. There was the overall flexibility of the backbone along with the ability to deep relaxation. Well, both these skills are available by yoga exercise.

Yoga is similar to the healthy nutrition. If you use it correctly in the optimal quantity, it will lead to unmatched physiological as well as psychological health. And this eventually reflects into your life, improving its overall quality. However, if you are probably trying to carry out the whole thing in yoga exercise instantly, the outcome could be comparable to striking random unusual postures.

It will be the motionless body along with the quiet mind (accomplished both in asana as well as in pauses between all of them) which is the fundamental factors for starting the technique of unprompted treatment of the system.

In daily life, the conscious mind is continually associated with the steps involved in socializing with the outside world and by no means stays vacant. This emptiness or silence of mind can solely take place in the performance of asana in line with Sutra 46, chapter II.

By some estimation, yoga in the USA is now a most dynamically developing form of physical activity. Here is the diagram which reflects that dynamic.

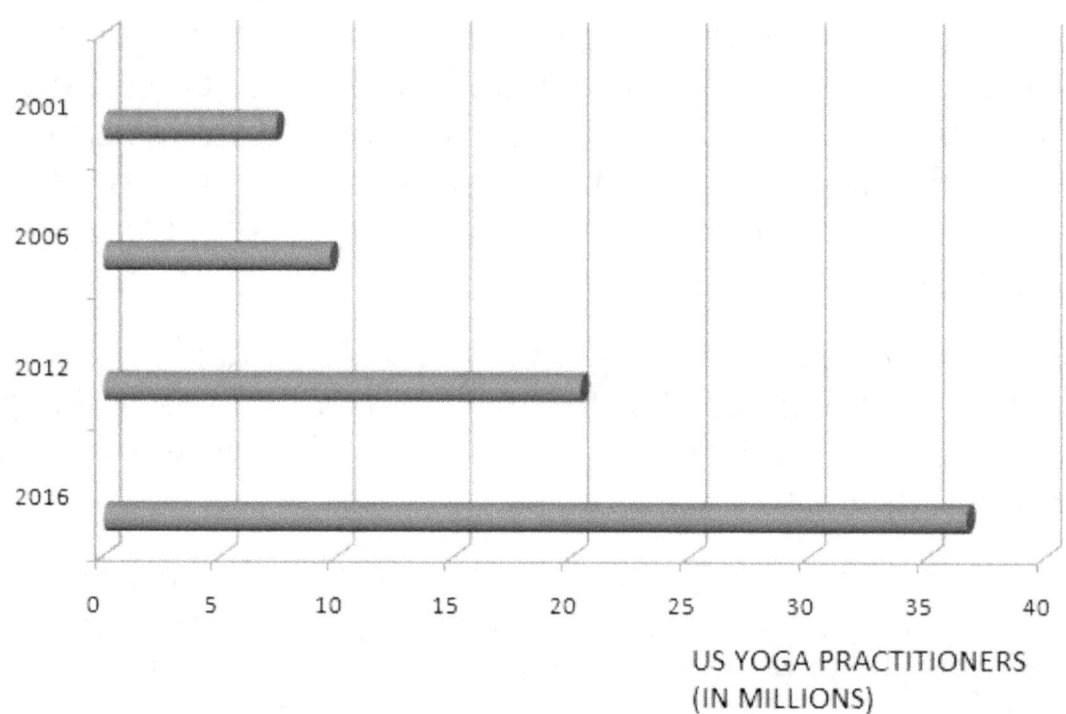

US YOGA PRACTITIONERS
(IN MILLIONS)

The approach of a person of the western mentality to yoga contains a drastic and rather dangerous mistake. Ancient texts do not mean the direct strong-willed control regarding the asana performance or meditation.

By its character, yoga is the ability of indirect control of the functional psychosomatic parameters (both controlled and automatic) using setting up specific conditions in both the entire body as well as the mind.

Definition of PSYCHOSOMATIC: of, relating to, concerned with, or involving both mind and body

We are going to look at the following instance. Eating is essential for surviving. Having acquired the cash, you can easily get the food, carry it home and even likely prepare it, arrange the table and sit down, get your hands on the food, put them into the mouth, gnaw and eat it. These would be your personal actions. However, what else could you do with the ingested food? Almost nothing, no more direct manipulations are feasible. The entire body further processes the meals alone, without your control. While the digestive breakdown of the food goes on, it gets to be self-regulating.

It is far from being smart to interrupt the means of breaking down the food. Through the existence of evolution, natural operations are characterized by their high level of effectiveness as well as autonomy from conscious control.

This instance is entirely congruent with classical or traditional yoga just as well. Yoga constantly was and is still the art of an indirect realignment. I only create conditions that my system by itself has led to the proper order. This order is known under the name of homeostasis. It is a hidden thing. We "learn" about its existence just after the appearance of disorder.

In traditional yoga, your body takes on asana, and the consciousness is virtually turned off not becoming involved with the process. The sequencing of poses, in the beginning, has no special meaning as it is defined according to the level of health and flexibility.

The irrelevant complication is not needed in yoga practice in any way. It is energy-consuming, dangerous, and not suitable for the proper yogic state of consciousness.

Classical Yoga Centers around Patanjali's Yoga Sutras.

"Asana is reached at the termination of effort or concentration on the infinite"

- «Yoga Sutras of Patanjali»

Sutras of Patanjali are a metaphorical explanation of the algorithm of traditional yoga practice. Such kind of yoga leads to the clearing and regeneration of your system. Then your contacts with outside world become optimal, as well as cooperation between your consciousness and sub-consciousness.

Sūtra (Sanskrit sū´tra), literally means a rope or thread that holds things together, and more metaphorically refers to an aphorism (or line, rule, formula), or a collection of such aphorisms in the form of a manual.

There are 196 Sutras of Patanjali. They are divided into eight 'limbs'. Practice on the physical level is only one of these parts. The name of this particular limb is asana. When you master your physical practice, you will be capable of learning other sides of yoga.

Patanjali is known as the father of yoga. He defines yoga as the cessation of recognition with the mental wandering. The first of Sutras is "Yoga is now." And this conception is not as simple as it sounds. Actually, achieving the now is challenging task.

Benefits of Yoga Practice

Practicing classical yoga always leads to recovery of the whole body system. That's why traditional yoga technique is a unique one. We consider such kind of yoga is a psychosomatic maintenance installed in the particular practice.

You could step by step rehab your physical and psychic health with the help of yoga. Of course, the result depends on your current stage and your age too. In theory, you could be regained from the weak position. But in real life, we always meet some difficulties. For instance, as a beginner, you need some adaptation period. Most likely, you will see results of practice only after that period.

Practice is a special "tempering" in the "fire" of yoga. When your body and your mind get ready, the siddhi appear.

Siddhi *(Sanskrit: siddhiḥ) is a Sanskrit word that literally means "perfection," "accomplishment," "attainment," or "success." It is also used as a term for spiritual power (or psychic ability).*

Rather than specifying their entire list, we will consider only one of them, "power." It is acquired only via long-term and quality practice of yoga.

We won't reside definition of every siddhi here. However, you should keep in your mind that any of these powers could be earned only by long-established and qualitative yoga practice.

There are too many variants how this power can influence practitioner's life. For example, you can notice that all issues you have met during nearest past are solved in the best of the possible way. Well, you should make a difference here. Your needs do not always coincide with your wishes. In fact, often they are opposite to each other. Your "power" doesn't support every dream generated by your mind.

You don't need too much time to get benefits of yoga poses. Yoga is an especial practice scheduled as part of your day which helps you to provide a high-grade life. Mentioned above power also impacts on relations with your family, friends, colleagues. The practicing person isn't in need of any sort of support anymore. It's opposite situation now. You become a source of calmness and energy for all people around you.

When you achieve some level of inner peace, you may notice that the favorable outcome in any affair relies solely on the quality of your calmness. Probably, you have already heard about benefits of brain work in alpha rhythm. So, throughout your practice, you are in alpha rhythm mostly.

Usually, your internal power directs situation in a right way even if the prognosis was adverse.

Traditional yoga improves the well-being of any person appreciably. If you are naturally healthy and well balanced emotionally, you still should practice gaining additional benefits and new opportunities.

General Guidelines

It is very special and positive ritual when you have woken up early in the morning then take your place on the mat and start practice. At some point in time, you start to feel your body entirely. You become a whole with your body, which bends and flows itself. All it happens without opposing, but with some primal pleasure. The ordinal thinking process is substituted by the inner silence, the rest, and the clarity. You get a positive impulse, and you keep it through the whole day long. You feel happy without particular reasons. You do not feel weariness, anxiety, irritation. You could build everything, to what you are capable on the base of your inner power.

The best time for yoga is precisely in the morning. If possible, don't postpone your practice to the evening.

Despite the similarity of all people, each one of us has his age, anthropometrical indicators, and health status. Certainly, you have also your natural level of flexibility. Due to a proper yoga practice, you can reach your limit, but it has never been the purpose of yoga. Yoga is not about development your acrobatic abilities. The value of the practice is something bigger. There is something like freedom from your mental vanity.

Thus, all-inclusive yoga recipe doesn't exist. You should master your practice personally individually. Your persistent attempts to force the body to complicated poses performing will result in injuries and regress in practice. So, the presence of experienced instructor is strongly recommended.

As a beginner you will probably go through the next several levels:

- Physical and psychological adaptation;

- Mastering a deep mental and physical relaxation;

- Creating an effective regimen of self-adjustment;

- Trying on advanced poses and techniques;

There should not be any discomfort during entering, holding, or exiting asana. It's a cornerstone of classical yoga. With the relaxation of your body and mind, all sensations pass out of sight. The intensity of practice remains within the typical range of routine activities, like walking, cleaning house, working on the computer, etc.

How actually should beginner execute an asana in a physical part? You should simply do asana. Just do it without impatience, or an expectation of result or excessive aspiration to make better, without any desire to do as in the picture.

To relax all muscles, you should run through the whole body with your attention. However, Sutras tell us just about the concentration on the infinity. So, how can you do that? The focus on the infinity means merely disengagement, not thinking about anything. And your inner silence is possible in deep relaxation of both mind and body.

To kick things off, when it comes to yoga as long as doing this will not affect your pose, shut your eyes. Seeing your surroundings while practicing is not OK. Closing your eyes has the added benefit of allowing you to avoid focusing on external things around you, which can aid in preventing you from concentrating on the senses. These static poses are used exactly for that very reason in order to release consciousness from the ordinary "contents."

When this is achieved, the solution has been found. The focus is solely on the body and not anything external, so there should be nothing binding or distracting you.

Mastering in asana means that your consciousness falls and the mental process becomes rarer. Along with this, the body starts to sink spontaneously in the form, "flowing down" to its absolute for today limit of flexibility.

You see, you should not do asana. You should simply be in asana! But the real comprehension of this trick and its implementation may cost a lot of time and efforts.

Performing asana correctly means to do so without any deception in you, or excessive diligence, and desire. Your will cannot change base properties of psychosomatics and processes in life support system.

For those who are just beginning, time of being in asana is mattered. It's an individual factor. There are signs in the body and mind that will tell you when to exit asana. Once you begin to feel these odd or uncomfortable sensations, you should immediately exit asana to avoid harming or injuring yourself. If you feel discomfort, or any abnormal sensations the moment you enter asana, this is a sign that your pose is too difficult for your expertise (or lack thereof) and that you should choose a more comfortable one. Unusual sensations can also be a sign that you have some possible injury or mental blockage making itself known.

Stretching asana may be repeated thrice in a row. If you are doing everything correctly, your body will effortlessly bend to the level attained the previous time and will continue to "flow" to a new provisional limit. Contrarily, if you find yourself struggling to hold poses, you most likely have some sort of unconscious mental blockage preventing you from advancing, or you have reached your current physical limitations of body's flexibility.

Other signals to exit emanate from the circulatory system, where you may experience burning, heavy breathing, numbness, and swelling during some positions. You may also experience pulsation in some areas of your body. If pulsation occurs in the same areas during different poses, then it may be a sign that you are injuring some blood vessels, or it is a symptom of underlying circulatory issues that you were unaware of.

Your exit from asana should be calm, flowing, without sensations and at ease, mentally and physically. To exit properly, allow your body to loosen naturally, almost straightening in the way a stress ball would after you squeeze it. If you any discomfort after exiting asana, pause and let it discontinue before entering the next posture.

When you perform the pose, make sure to hold it for the proper amount of time, so your body gets the maximum benefit from it. When you begin to feel certain symptoms and sensations, it is an indication that you should end or switch postures.

One vital part of asana is to remember that hurting yourself is contradictory to ahimsa. The fundamental principle of the classical yoga is a not producing damage to the own body. Pain is a signal of injury, so you should avoid pain.

After some practice in asana, you will keep to a minimum the number of muscles involved as well as the intensity of their work. The valuable exposure time in asana lasts from the moment when you are motionless until the coming of sensations. When you begin to feel these sensations, stop the asana.

You should not feel discomfort during asana. You should not sweat heavily; feel pain, or any other unusual sensations. The foundation of yoga is not to hurry, but to relax in a way that one cannot in daily life. Asana requires a particular state of mind as well, and it is very much a holistic process, though you may not notice this at first.

Yoga requires holding certain poses; in fact, this is the foundation of yoga. It is using your body's weight and parts; it is the moving and crossing of limbs, and changing the body so that you maximize benefits received from gravity.

Tough poses should only be done by those who can do them without exerting too much effort, both physical and mental. You should be able to maintain a relaxed state of mind while doing asana.

For those just beginning yoga, the first step is to direct one's gaze towards the body. The eyes are typically the easiest way in which you can focus. Eyes should remain closed during practice since almost everyone receives information visually and visual stimulation can great affect your ability to relax the mind significantly. With closed eyelids the eyeballs habitually keep reflex moving around or shaking.

Shavasana is the recommended choice for beginners, one should be able to relax the eyeballs in such a way that they no longer spontaneously move or twitch at random. Oftentimes the eyes will move to find the most comfortable position. The eye orbits start to perceive weight, occasionally lukewarm, and the mind relaxed sets on this sector. However, the moment something catches the attention of the eye, it will strain again and move around like they normally do. This is why it is important that one practice relaxing the eyes so that the mind can relax as well and the mental activity slows down.

After accomplishing total relaxation of muscles in asana, the human body does only work that is needed. If you avoid making your posture better despite the negative sensations, there is no risk of having traumas.

These descriptions will be applicable only for those people whose natural flexibility allows to perform all that poses rather freely. It is not worth even reading of these descriptions in the initial phase of mastering yoga for those who are capable of reproducing the form of asana only approximately. What sense does it make if the body is able to be bent in a position far from being similar to what is in the image? As the novice gets more practice and begins to grasp the technique, his body flexibility starts to grow in itself. The asana which did not resemble the original become to get more and more similar to that which is in the image. After this, texts can now be used as a form of guidance to the practice.

Corpse Pose (Savasana)

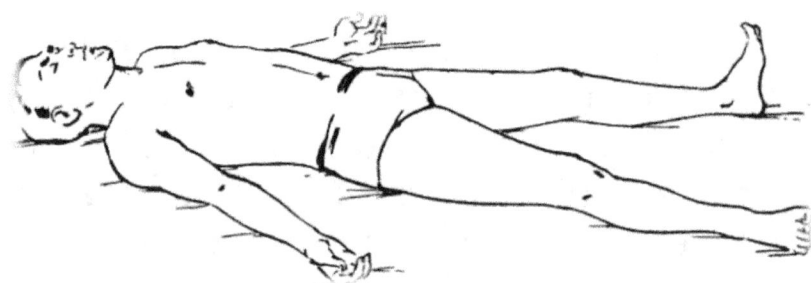

Bend your knees and sit on the floor, put both feet on the floor and recline backward on your forearms. Breathe in, then stretch the right leg slowly, do the same to the left leg pushing through the heels. Now both legs should be released with the groins softened. Ensure the legs are positioned at angles that are equal about the middle line of the torso. Also, take great care that both feet are turned out the same way. Now, the front pelvis should be narrowed, and the lower back should be softened but not flattened.

Reach for the ceiling with your arms perpendicular to the flooring. Oscillate gently from left to right, and then release your arms to the floor. Your arms should then be at angles that are equal about the middle of your body. Hands should be turned outwards.

Savasana serves the dual purpose of quieting the sense organ and the physical body. The wings of the nose, root of the tongue, channels of the inner ears and the bridge of the nose, which is between the eyebrows, should be softened. Release your eyes to the back of the head.

This pose should be maintained for at least 5 minutes for every half-hour of practice. To exit this pose, you should roll to one side (your right preferably) while exhaling once. Then two or three breaths should be taken. Your hands should press against your floor, and your body should be lifted.

If the relaxation is indeed profound, there is possible a little quivering of the muscle felt in Shavasana. This quivering seems like ripples of water. Usually, it starts on the left of the face if you are right handed. This quivering then extends to the right part of the body. It may then lead to a spontaneous dance of the muscles. This appearance is one of the ways by which mental stress is relieved, so there is nothing to fear or react.

Seated Forward Bend (Paschimottanasana)

Asana should always be done like breathing or walking. There should be no endeavor made to make them better. If no sensation is felt, then the asana is done perfectly.

Therefore, Paschimottanasana can be held for a long time. The body will jack-knife, and the torso will lie flat on straightened legs. This position won't give you any sensations which will be similar to Shavasana. You might feel tiny echoes of musculoskeletal movements, but they won't disturb the calmness of your mind.

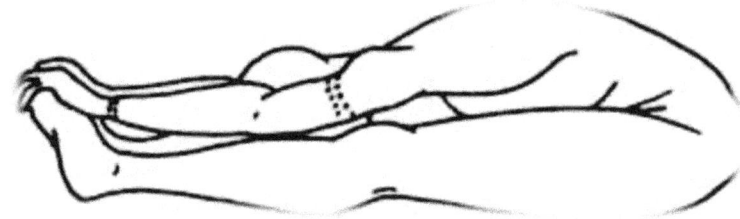

Support your buttocks on a blanket that is folded while you are seated with your legs in front of you. Your heels should be used to press actively. The top thighs should be pulled in a little, and then pushed to the ground. Your palms should then be pressed to the floor beside the hips, and the top part of the sternum should be lifted to the roof as the top thighs are brought down.

If you can, use your hands to take the side of your feet with your thumbs on the soles of your feet and your elbows fully extended. But if this is not possible, then you can loop a strap around the soles of your foot while holding the strap firmly.

When you wish to go further, don't use force to pull yourself into a forward bend. You should always lengthen the front torso into that pose while keeping your head raised. If your feet are being held, your elbows should be bent to the sides and lifted away from the floor. If the strap is being held, then your grip should be lightened, and your hands should be walked forward while your arms should be kept long.

As you inhale, you should lift and lengthen your front torso a little. As you make each exhalation, you should release a bit more into the forward bend. This way, the body oscillates, lengthens a little with the every breath.

This pose should be maintained for about one to three minutes. In order to come up, you should lift your torso away from your thighs.

Never try to force yourself into a forward bend especially when you are sitting on the floor. When coming forward, as soon as the space between your navel and pubis is shortening, you should stop, lift up slightly and lengthen again. At first, because you have tightness in the back of your legs, your forward bend will not go far forward and might look like sitting straight up.

Cobra Pose (Bhujangasana)

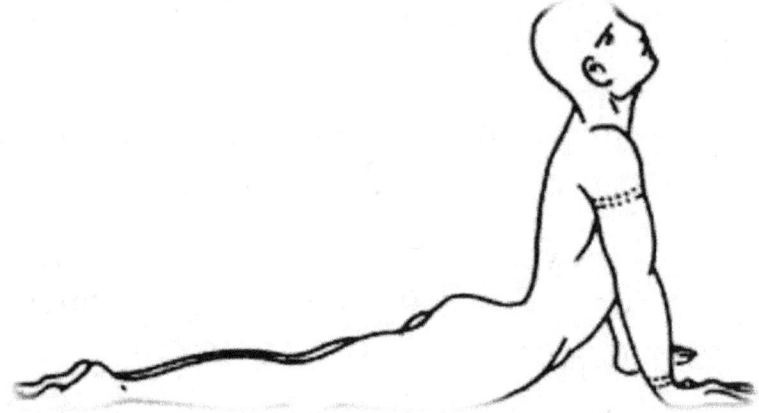

Lie on your tummy. Straighten your legs back and place the tips of your feet on the floor. Your hands spread out under your shoulders while your elbows are embraced into your body.

Your thighs, pubis and the tips of your feet should be pressed firmly to the ground.

Breathe in and then gradually straighten out your hands to lift your chest off the floor. Ensuring that you do not go beyond the height within which you can maintain a link with your pubis and legs. The tailbone should be pressed towards the pubis while the pubis itself is lifted towards the direction of the navel. Ensure the hip points are contracted firmly but not too much to avoid it toughening the backsides

Place the shoulder blades firmly against the back, pushing out the side ribs forward. Lift the shoulder blades through the top of the sternum while ensuring that the forefront ribs are not pushed forward. This way you prevent it from hardening the lower back region. Share the backbend equally all through the whole spine.

Maintain this posture for about 15 to 30 seconds, breathing effortlessly. Breathe out and discharge the back to the floor. Try not to do the backbend excessively. To discover the limit at which you can easily work without straining your back, release your hand from the floor for a split second so the height you will see will be the accurate extension you can comfortably work

Locust Pose (Salabhasana)

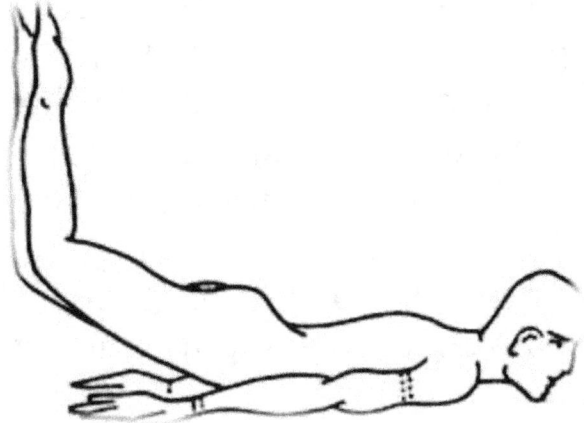

This pose might require you to cushion the floor beneath your pelvis and ribs with a blanket. After the padding, you then lie on your stomach while keeping your hands on the sides of your torso, with your palms raised up while your forehead remains on the floor. Place your big toes to face each other so that they can internally pivot your thighs, firmly place your backside so that your coccyx is pressed toward your pubis.

Breathe out and lift your head, upper middle, hands, and legs from the floor. Then, you rest on your lower ribs, stomach, and front pelvis. Place your backside firmly and try to reach through to your legs, starting from the heels to stretch the back legs, then through the bases of the big toes. Ensure the big toes are turned in the direction of each other.

Keep your arm raised parallel to the floor and extend back actually using your fingertips. Envision there's weight pushing down on the backs of the upper arms, and push up toward the roof against this opposition. Keep your scapulas pressed solidly into your back.

Look forward or somewhat upward, being mindful so as not to bulge your chin forward and crux the back of your neck. Ensure the base end of the skull is lifted while the back of the neck is kept long.

Maintain this posture about 30 to 60 seconds and then breath out and discharge at the same time. Breathe in and out a couple of time and try to repeat these 1 or 2 times if you wish. Starters often find it a bit challenging to lift the torso and the legs in this posture. Start the pose with your hands lying on the floor, a somehow back from the shoulders, nearer to your waist. Breathe in and gradually push your hands against the floor to help lift the upper middle. At that point, keep the hands set up as you do the posture, or after a couple of breaths, once you have ensured the chest is lifted up, swing them once more into the position explained above. Concerning the legs, you can practice the pose with the legs raised off the floor one at a time. For instance, you have to lift the left leg off the floor for about half a minute and then do same for the right leg if you want to hold the pose for one minute.

Shoulder stand (Sarvangasana)

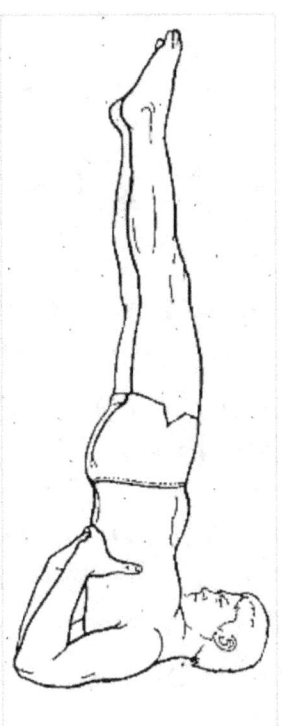

Lay down on your back, arms alongside your upper-body. Then bend your knees and put your feet on the floor with the heels close to the buttocks. Breathe out, press your arms firmly against the floor and lift your feet from the floor.

Keep your upper arms on the mat and stretch your palms against the reins. Raise your torso to the position relatively perpendicular to the floor.

Breathe in and bring your thighs in line with upper body keeping heels close to sitting bones. It's time now to unbend your knees.

To exit from the pose, breathe out and bend your knees again. Then roll your back down into the ground. Be careful and keep your head on the floor all the time.

Start with 30 seconds holding this asana. Add 5 or 10 seconds every time you practicing. Soon you will be able to stay for 3 minutes in Sarvangasana without any discomfort.

Plow Pose (Halasana)

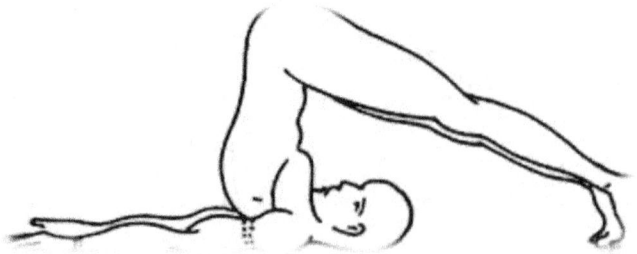

From Sarvangasana, breathe out and twist from the hip joints to gradually bring down your toes to the floor beneath and above your head. As much as you can, keep your middle region vertical and your legs completely straightened.

Keep your top thighs and tailbone raised toward the roof while your toes are kept on the floor. Draw your inward groins deep into the pelvis. Envisage that your middle region is dangling from the height of your crotches. Keep on bringing your chin far from your sternum and soften your throat.

You can keep on pressing your hands against the back of your middle region, while you press the back of your upper arm down. As another variant, you can discharge your hands from your back and straighten arms behind you on the floor, opposite the legs. Clip the hands and press the arms down on the support as you lift the thighs toward the roof.

Halasana is performed after Sarvangasana within 1 to 5 minutes. To release yourself from the pose, bring your hands back to your back once more, lift once again into Sarvangasana while breathing out, then move down to your back. In this particular pose, there is a possibility of you overstretching the neck by pulling the shoulders too far from the ears. In as much as the shoulder tops ought to push down into the support, they should also be lifted marginally toward the ears to hold the back of the neck and throat. You should open the sternum by keeping the shoulder blades firm against the back.

Bow Pose (Dhanurasana)

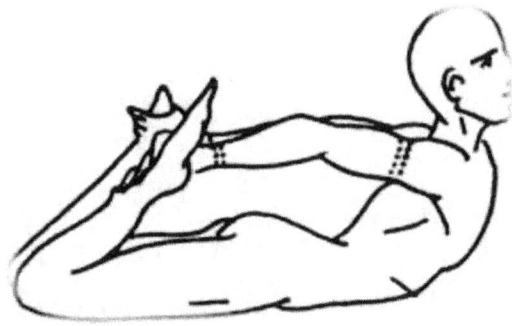

Lie on your tummy with your hands along your body and your palms placed up. Breathe out and flex your knees, bringing your heels as close as you can to your back side. Grab your lower legs using your hands through the back. Note that it must not be tops of your feet. Ensure your knees are not much wider than the breadth of your hips and keep your knees hip width throughout the period of this pose.

Breathe in and firmly lift your heels from your bottom and in the meantime, lift your thighs from the floor. This action will have the impact of pulling your upper torso and your head away from the floor. Tunnel the tailbone down toward the floor, and hold your back muscles soft. Keep lifting the heels and the thighs higher, while keeping the shoulder blades pressed against your back to be able to open your heart. Maintain the shoulder tops drawn away from your ears and look ahead.

Press your stomach against the floor. This act will make breathing to be difficult. However, you have to keep breathing and breathe more into the back of your torso. You do not have to stop breathing.

Maintain this pose for about 20-30 seconds. Free yourself gradually as you breathe out and breathe for a couple of times while you are rest.

Feel free to repeat this pose for 1 or 2 times more if you wish.

Hero Pose (Virasana)

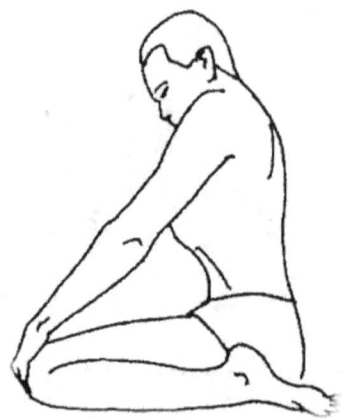

Go down on your knees on the ground and use the blanket as support between your calves and thighs if needed. Ensure your thighs are kept at an angle of 90° to the floor, and your inner knees are touching each other. Keep your feet separated from each other, a little bit wider than the knees and the tops of the feet should be kept flat on the ground. Then, you keep your big toes to face each other inwards while pressing the tops of both legs evenly on the ground.

Breathe out and sit midway, with your upper body kept a bit forward. Then, try sitting in between your feet.

Place a thick book or block in between the legs and use them to raise your buttocks if they do not comfortably rest on the floor. Keep a space of about the width of the thumbs between the inner heels and the outer hips. Press the heads of the thigh bones into the ground with your palms. Then keep your hands in your laps with palms down.

Place your shoulder blades strongly against the back ribs and straight your torso, like a fighter proud of his victories. Pull your collarbones slightly down and backward. Discharge the shoulder blades far from the ears. Protract the tailbone into the floor to hold the back-middle region of your body.

Initially, remain in this pose for about 30-60 seconds. Elongate your stay bit by bit up to 5 minutes. To release yourself, press your hands into the floor and raise your backside up a bit above the heels. Keep your ankles crossed underneath and sit backward on the feet and the ground. Then extend your legs before you. It might feel great to skip your knees here and there a couple of times on the floor.

Boat Pose (Navasana)

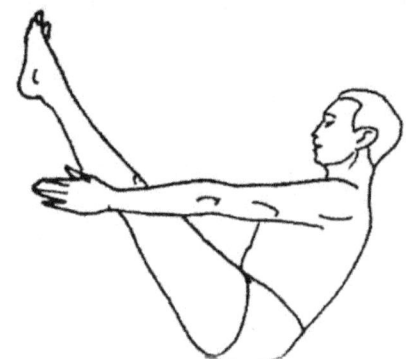

Take sit-on-the-floor with your legs straight before you and keep your hands firmly on the ground somewhat behind your hips with the fingers pointing towards the feet. Then lean back slightly. Make sure your back does not round as you do this. Sit on the "support" of your two sitting bones and tailbone.

Breathe out and twist your knees, then try raising your feet off the ground, so that the thighs are at an angle of about 45-50 degrees to the floor. Protract your tailbone into the floor and lift your pubis toward your navel. Gradually straighten your knees where possible, lifting the tips of your toes a bit over the level of your eyes. However, remain with your knees bent if this is not feasible maybe just lifting the shins parallel to the floor.

Straight out your arms parallel to each other and the floor. If it isn't feasible, you can place the hands on the ground near your hips, or otherwise, you hold on to the back of the thighs.

In as much as your abdomen should be kept firm, it should not be allowed to get hard and thick. It should be kept as flat as possible. Breathe effortlessly. Initially, you can remain in this position for about 10-20 seconds. Step by step you should increases the duration of stay to 1 minute.

Discharge the legs with an exhalation and sit upright while you inhale. You can rehearse this posture occasionally throughout your day even while sitting on your seat.

Downward-Facing Dog (Adho Mukha Svanasana)

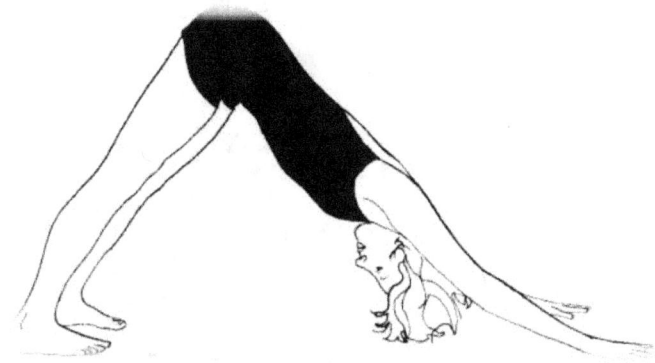

Get to the floor on your hands and knees. Your knees should be kept directly below your hips with your hands placed slightly onwards on your shoulders. Spread out your palms with your fingers turned out. Keep your toes under.

Breathe out and raise your knees above the ground. Initially, let the knees be kept bowed and the heels raised far from the floor. Then lift the sitting bones toward the roof. Breath out again and push your top thighs back and straighten your heels onto or down toward the floor. Straight out your legs.

Place your shoulder blades firmly against your back, then them wider and draw them toward the tailbone. Ensure the head is kept between the upper arms; never allow it to hang.

To come out, bend your knees to the floor while breathing out and rest.

Chair Pose (Utkatasana)

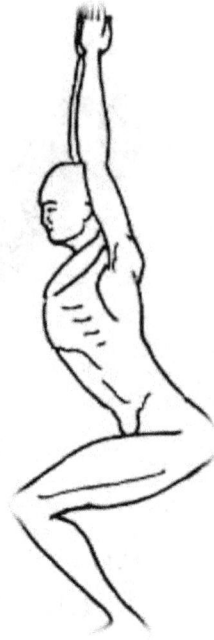

Stand with your feet together. Breathe in and raise your arms vertical to the ground. You can either join the palms or keep the arms parallel while the hands face inward.

Breathe out and bend your knees. You should keep your thighs as parallel to the floor as possible. Lean your upper body slightly forth until it stays at 90 degrees with the tops of the thighs. Ensure the inner thighs are parallel to each other and keep the heads of the thigh bones pressed toward the heels.

Maintain this position for about 30-60 seconds. To release yourself from this pose, make your legs straight while breathing in. Then breathe out and bring your arms back to your sides into the start position.

Eagle Pose (Garudasana)

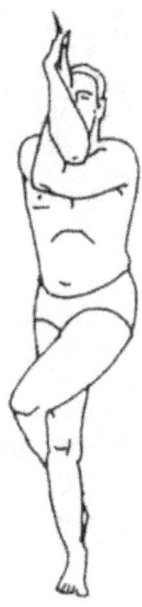

Stand with your feet together and with your knees bent slightly. Rise up your left foot and keep yourself balanced on the right foot. Then, you cross your left thigh over the right. Place your left toes pointed to the ground and kept the foot pressed back. After which you hook the top of the foot at the back of the lower right calf.

Straight out your arms. Then cross them in front of your torso in such a way that the right arm is kept above the left and then bend your elbows. Place the right elbow inside the crook of the left and maintain the forearm lifted vertically to the floor. Ensure that the back of your hands is facing each other.

Place your palms together. Ensure that the biggest finger of the right hand is passed in front of the little finger of the left hand and press the palms together as firmly as you can. Raise your elbows up and straight your fingers out to face the roof.

Maintain this position for about 15 to 30 seconds and release the legs and the arms and then stand in the start position. Go through the same process within the same time frame but your legs and arms inverted this time. As a beginner, you might have some difficulty to hook the lifted left leg behind the standing leg calf and keep it balanced on the standing foot.

For the first times, you might cross the legs and press the big toe of the leg foot instead of hook it. Keep the big toe pressed against the floor to help you hold it in balance.

Extended Side Angle (Utthi Parsvakonasana)

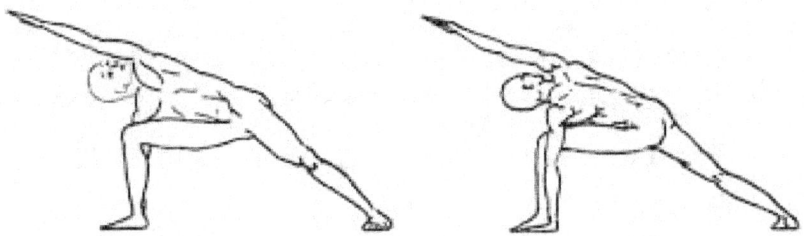

Stand with your feet to about 3.5 to 4 feet apart. Lift your arms parallel to the floor and let them be reached out actively to the sides. Your scapulas should be placed wide, and your palms kept down. Place the left of your foot a bit at a right angle to the right of your foot.

Keep the right heel aligned with the left heel. Roll the left hip slightly forth, toward the right, but rotate your upper body back to the left side.

Breathe out and curve the right knee in such a way the shin is placed vertically to the floor. You should bring the right thigh to be parallel to the ground.

Straighten out your left arm to face the ceiling and then twist your left palm in such a way that it will face towards the direction of your head. Then breathe in and reach the arm over the back of your left ear with your palm down. Redirect your head to face your left arm and discharge your right shoulder far from your ear.

Breathe out as you keep your left heel placed to the ground and lay your right upper body down as close as possible to the top of the right thigh. Keep your palms pressed on the ground just outside of your right foot.

Maintain this position for about 30-60 seconds and breathe in to come up. Most beginners often experience two challenges in this asana.

One of the problems is their inability to keep the back of their heels firm to the ground as they bend their front knee into this pose. The solution to this problem is to support your back heel against a wall. Imagine that you are pushing the wall away from you with your heel.

The other one is that they find it difficult to touch the fingertips of the lower hand once they are in this position. The solution for you is to rest your forearm on the top of the bent knee instead of trying to touch the ground.

Tree Pose (Vrksasana)

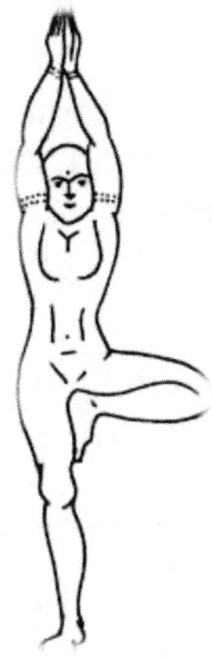

Stand with your feet together. Transfer your weight a bit more on the left foot and keep the inner side of your foot placed firmly on the floor and twisted your right knee. Use your right hand to reach out and hold your right ankle.

Your foot should be drawn up and placed the sole against the inner left thigh. Point your toes towards the floor and hold the right heel into the inner left groin. Clasp your palms together at heart.

Maintain this position for about 30-60 seconds. Breathe out and stand in the start position. Do the same asana within the same frame of time but with your legs reversed.

Conclusion

A lot of beginners fail to understand that total absence of something could be more valuable than its presence. This one is a primary reason why most of the novices overdo their asana practice, giving room to sensations of little pains which makes them feel that they are doing useful work.

During every asana practice, even at intermissions between them, we delegate powers to the system, to change and control the course of events. Everything else, such as feeling better, improved flexibility, relief of stress is results of this delegation.

'Action by not action' as described by Patanjali is the central principle of classical yoga. Traditional yoga is a gentle management of initial conditions. As a result, the system works in itself in a direction useful to it and hence helpful to me. Any physical or mental activity constructed from the beginning to the end on personal efforts and self-control is not classical yoga!

Combining mental silence with asana practice is partly a meditation, with all the effects flowing from it. The word 'partly' is used because for you to meditate you need not to move for an extended period which is impossible in most of the yoga poses.

We have already mentioned study 2016 about yoga in the US earlier in this book. There are few curious stats, which I would like to comment.

1.   There are almost 14 million yoga practitioners over the age of 50 in the US.

This one looks like pretty good evidence of positive impact of yoga practice on your active longevity. And it is worthy, isn't it?

2.   75% of yoga practitioners also engage in other physical exercises including running, group sports, weightlifting, and cycling.

Yoga teachers are seven times more likely to practice martial arts than is the average US adult.

As you can see, yoga is only a part of the physical culture for the biggest part of practitioners. Actually, I consider yoga practice as an excellent recovery from sports stress.

3.   98% of practitioners consider themselves to be beginner or intermediate level practitioners.

It was a key reason for writing this book. So, it is also a good cause to say one more time "thank you" for purchasing my book! I hope that you have enjoyed it. You should start your practice as soon as you can.

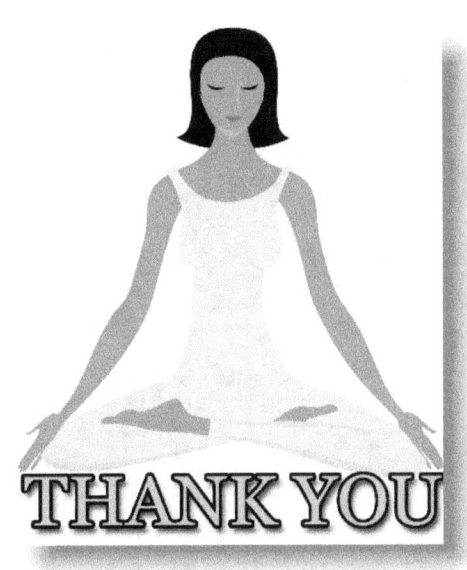